Yellow Gerbera

Little Book of Affirmations

J L Herald

Yellow Gerbera

Copyright © 2024 JL Herald

All rights reserved.

This book or any portion thereof may not be reproduced or used in any manner whatsoever without the express written permission of the copyright owner, except for the use of brief quotations in a book review.

First Printed 2024
by Yellow Gerbera Publishing
Australia

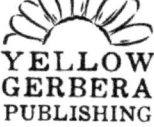

Cover Design © JL Herald 2024
with artwork by TheDigitalCraftCo

ISBN: 978-0-6459915-67 (paperback)
Website: http://www.JLHerald-poet.com

This little book
is for you to take with you
when the hamsters start spinning
and take hold of your head
to remind you those echoes
are not who you are
that you are worthy
and you deserve love

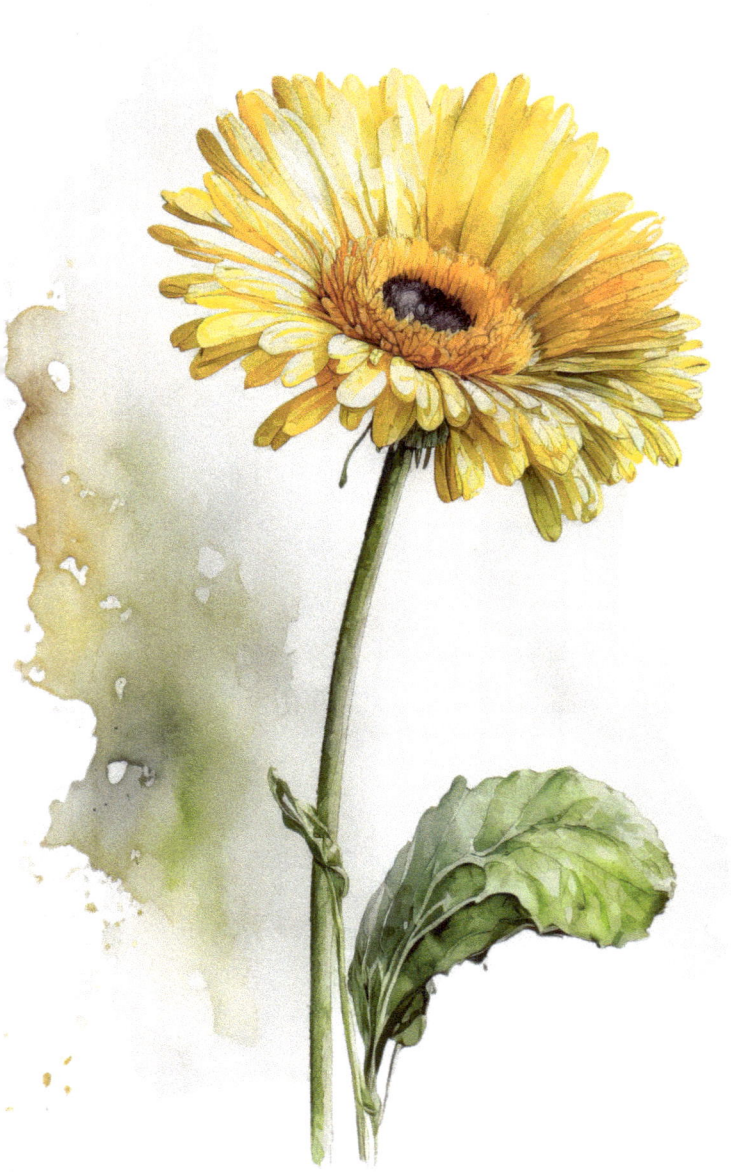

On a rocky stony cliff
overlooking the ocean blue
a little yellow gerbera grows
in a crack of dirt within the stone.

Buffeted by salty winds,
soaked by ocean waves
the little yellow gerbera holds on
quietly growing all alone.

It doesn't matter how strong the winds become
or how high the waves are storming
that little yellow gerbera keeps growing
its face towards the sun.

- Resilience -
toxic/empathy © 2024
JL Herald

This book provides positive affirmations for those recovering from toxic relationships.

This might be a familial relationship, friend relationship or romantic relationship. A relationship where you leave with your self-esteem in tatters, and questioning your self-worth and memory.

Any time you are feeling low, questioning yourself, wondering what you did that was wrong, remember the yellow gerbera.

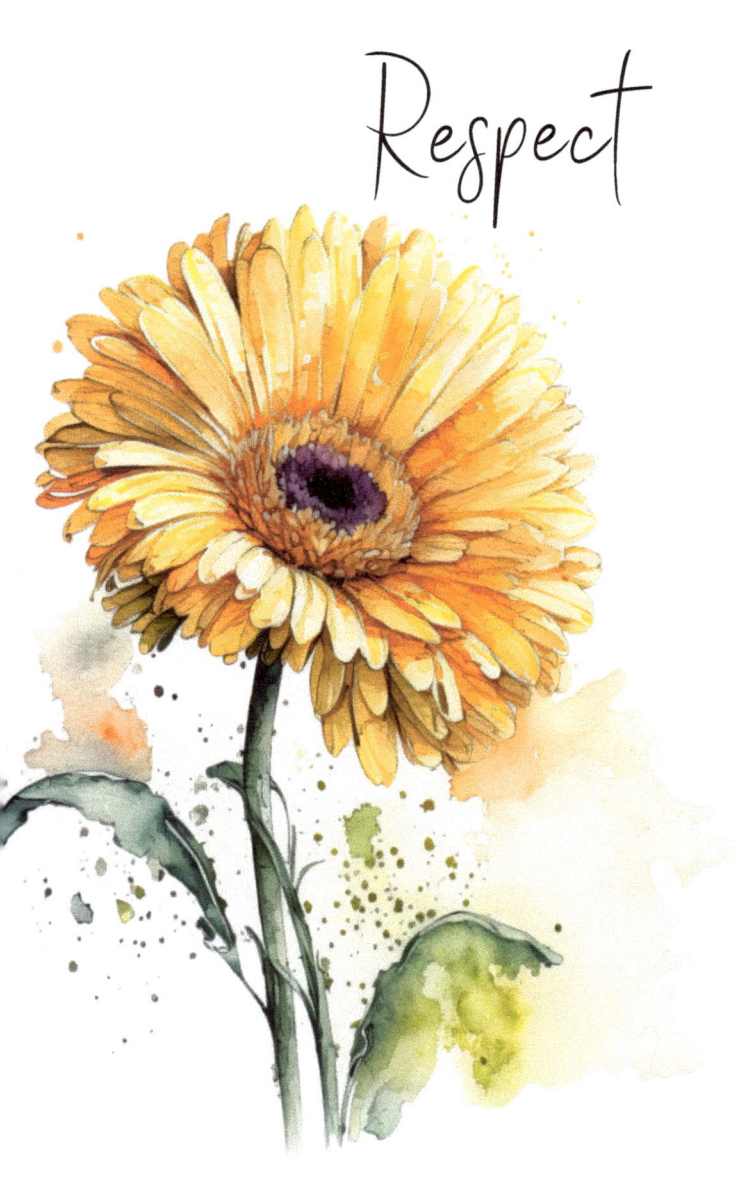
Respect

I deserve to always be treated with respect and dignity

I am not responsible for the choices other people make.

If they choose to threaten, intimidate, or belittle, I did not make them do it.

If someone cannot talk to me without getting angry, yelling, or blaming — then they do not respect me, and I do not have to continue being around them.

I do not have to accept being spoken to in a way that makes me the only one at fault.

If someone says that care about me, then they would feel horrified that their actions hurt me.

If they do not - that shows you who they are.

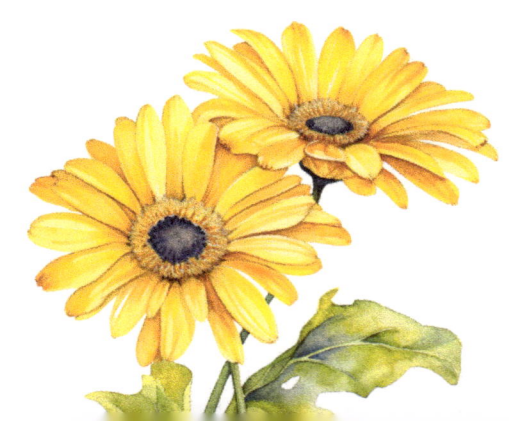

No-one has the right to take advantage of me.

If I chose to tell someone about private matters, and they tell others, they are not worth my time or effort.

People that expose my personal secrets are using my pain to further themselves, and do not respect me.

My ability to love is a reflection on me.

Their desire to hurt me is a reflection on them.

Love does not hurt you.

Love does not shame you.

Love does not make you feel small or worthless.

My hopes and dreams are valid and important.

Shaming them is not an act of love or respect

My voice is important.

I am allowed to express myself
and give my own opinion
without being scorned.

No.

I do not have to explain why.

I made mistakes too.

I own them, and the hurt that they created.

I will learn and grow and know that those mistakes made me human, and growth makes me worthy.

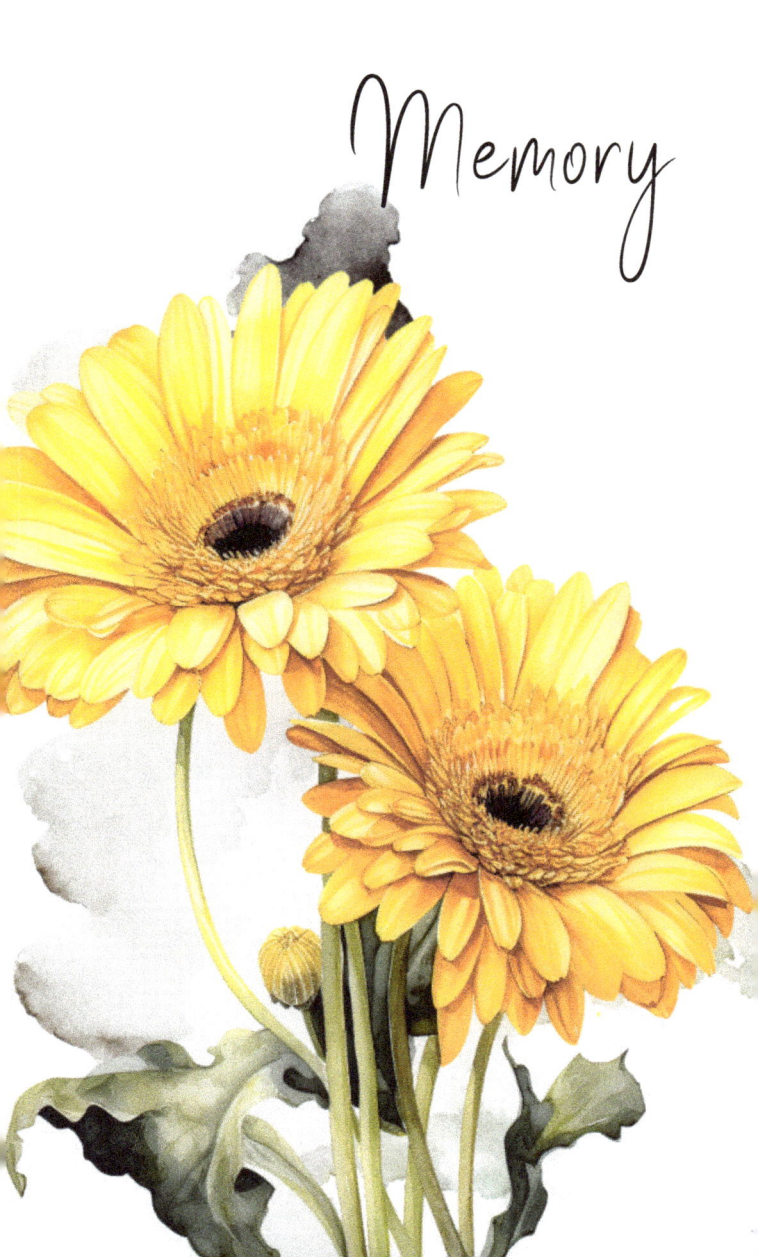

My memory is not up for discussion.

I know what happened.

I was there.

I can read.

I can see.

I can understand.

My reality is not dictated by someone who tells me the words I have in front of me are not real.

I trust my own mind.

I do not accept being lied to about what I know to be true.

I will hold strong to my memory and do not doubt that I know what reality is.

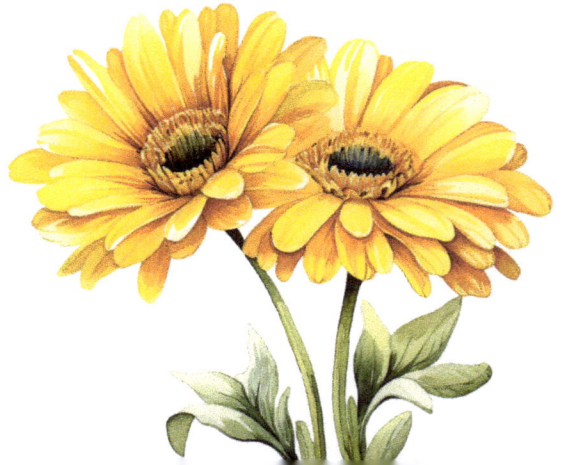

I do not have a mental disorder because I choose not to believe their mistruths.

I do not need another to validate and confirm what I know is real.

My memory is not leading me astray, the person making me doubt myself is.

I am not crazy.

I am in control of myself.

I choose myself, and that makes me strong.

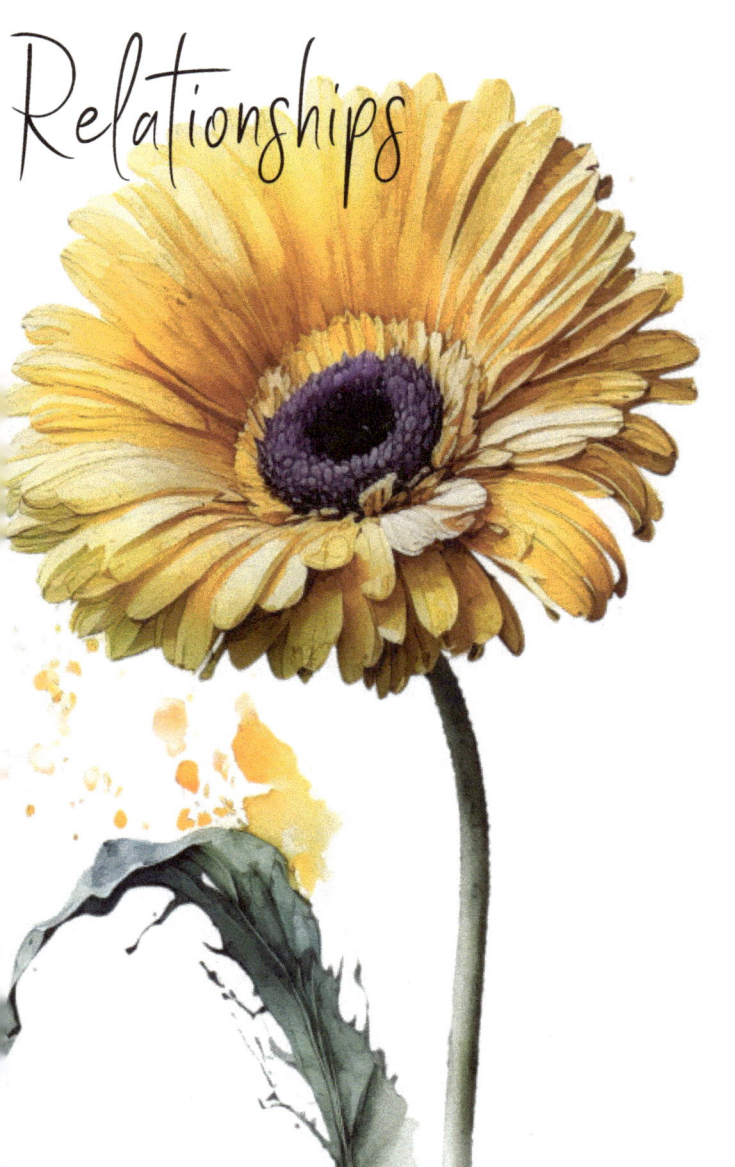
Relationships

I will create strong boundaries and hold to them.

Boundaries are there to ensure that I have healthy relationships.

I am attractive and can have happy and healthy relationships.

I cared even when they were hurting me.

That means I can love; I just gave it to someone that did not deserve it.

I am willing to walk away from toxic relationships.

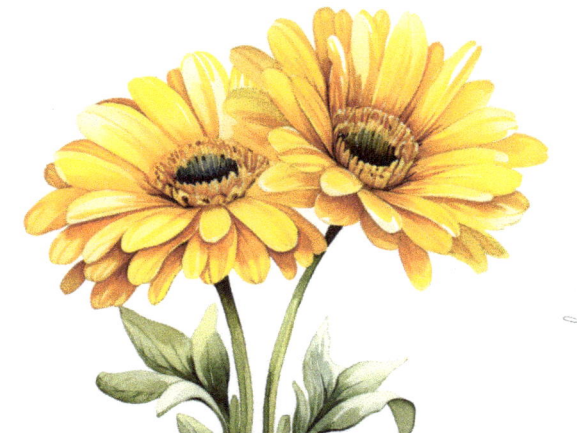

I know what toxic patterns look like, and choose to break free from them.

I will put in the effort to grow as a person, and open my heart for the possibilities of healthy relationships.

I made mistakes too.

I own them, and the hurt that they created.

I will learn and grow and know that those mistakes made me human, and growth makes me worthy.

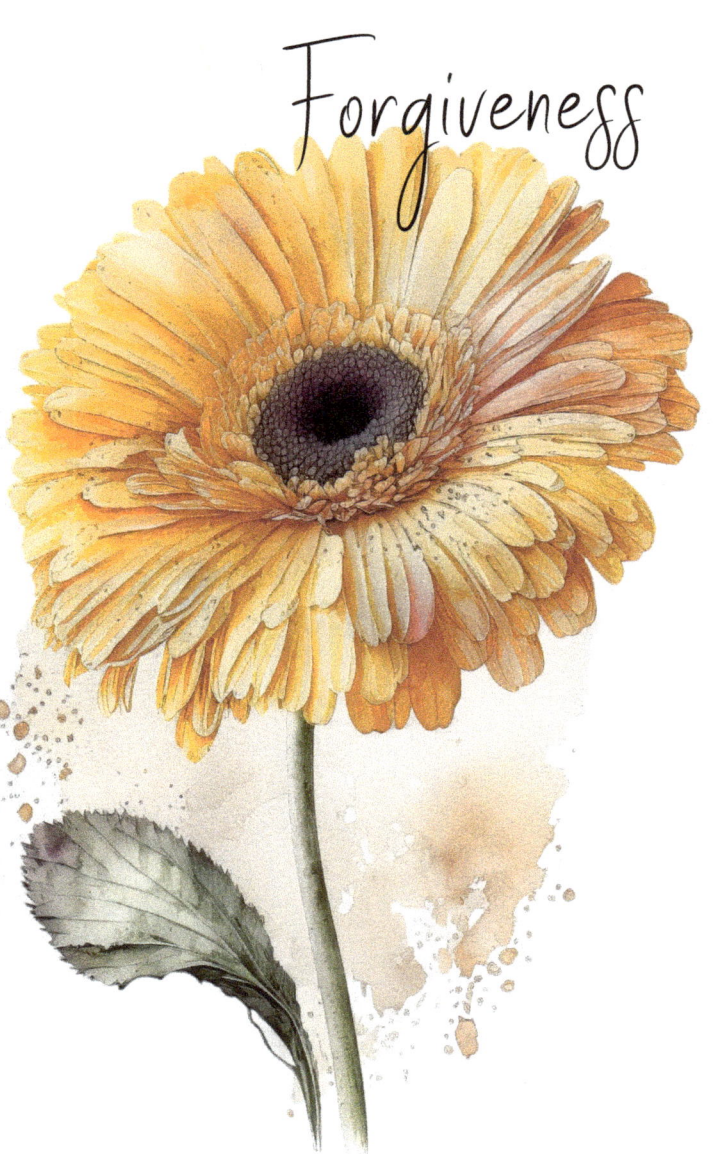

I forgive myself.

It is okay to let go of wanting an apology from those that have hurt me and refuse to take responsibility for their actions.

I do not have to forgive a person who has hurt me.

Forgiveness is about me.

I can choose to forgive someone and that is okay.

I can choose not to forgive them, and that is okay too.

Being hurt was not my fault.

I did not make them hurt me.

If I hurt someone, I will take responsibility for it, and apologise.

I will not become the person that hurt me.

I will release myself from toxic connections in my life

I am strong enough to choose
what is best for me

I am not defined by my past relationships.

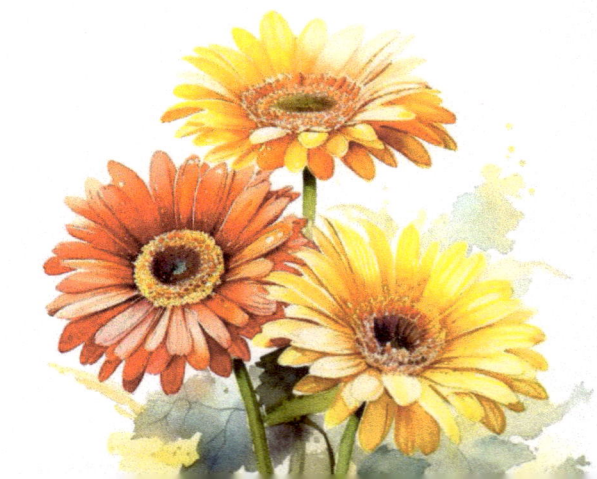

My happiness is within me, I control it.

I choose peace.

I choose to walk away from conflict.

I will make the changes I need.
I am empowered to be the
positive influence

I forgive myself for the mistakes that I made, and the red flags I chose not to see.

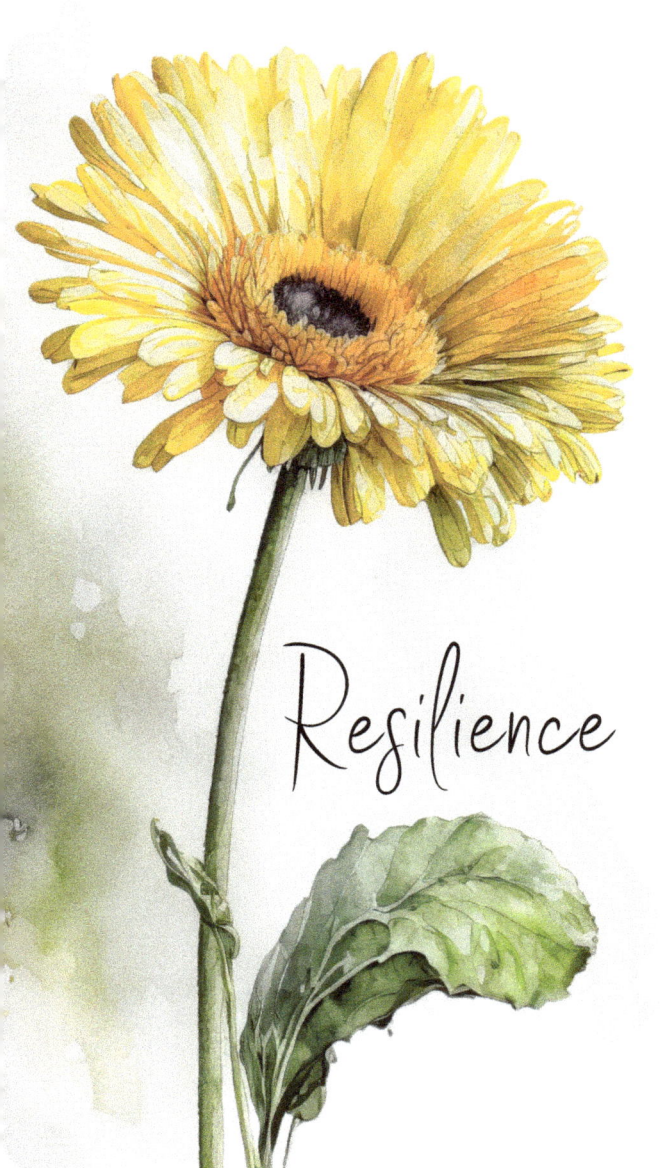

I am strong.

I may falter

But I refuse to fall

I may cry.

I may feel crazy.

I may fall apart.

I will survive and I will be stronger.

I will hold true to myself, even as they try to break me

I may feel battered and broken, but this is only temporary.

Being hurt was not my fault.
I did not make them hurt me.

I am not alone.

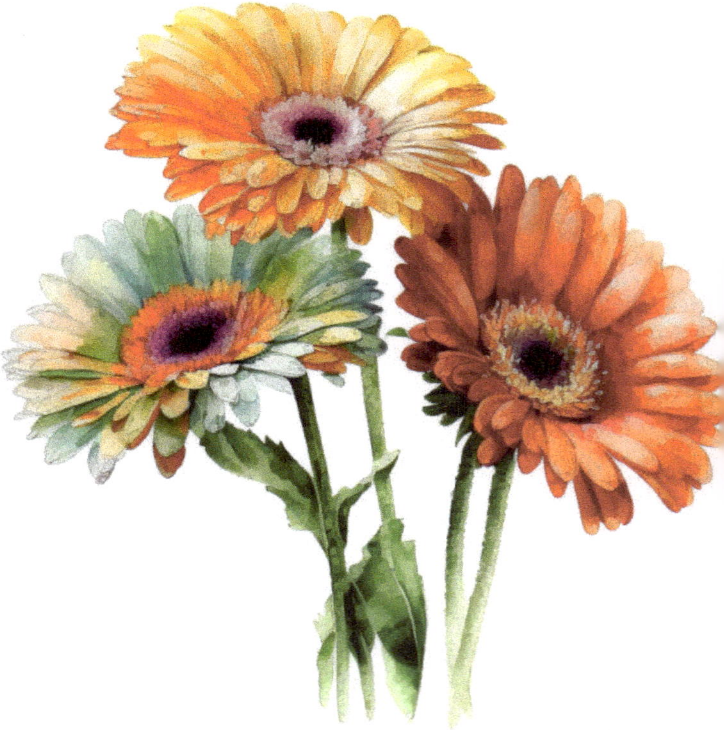

I am a survivor.

I am not a victim.

I have the right to say no when I do not like a situation and I am feeling uncomfortable, scared, or frightened.

I had challenges to overcome in the past.

They have made me resilient.

I am free to make my own choices, for my own goals.

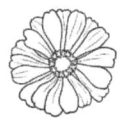

I can only control myself.

I cannot expect change in people that refuse to see an issue in what they do.

I will be my own light, and follow my own path.

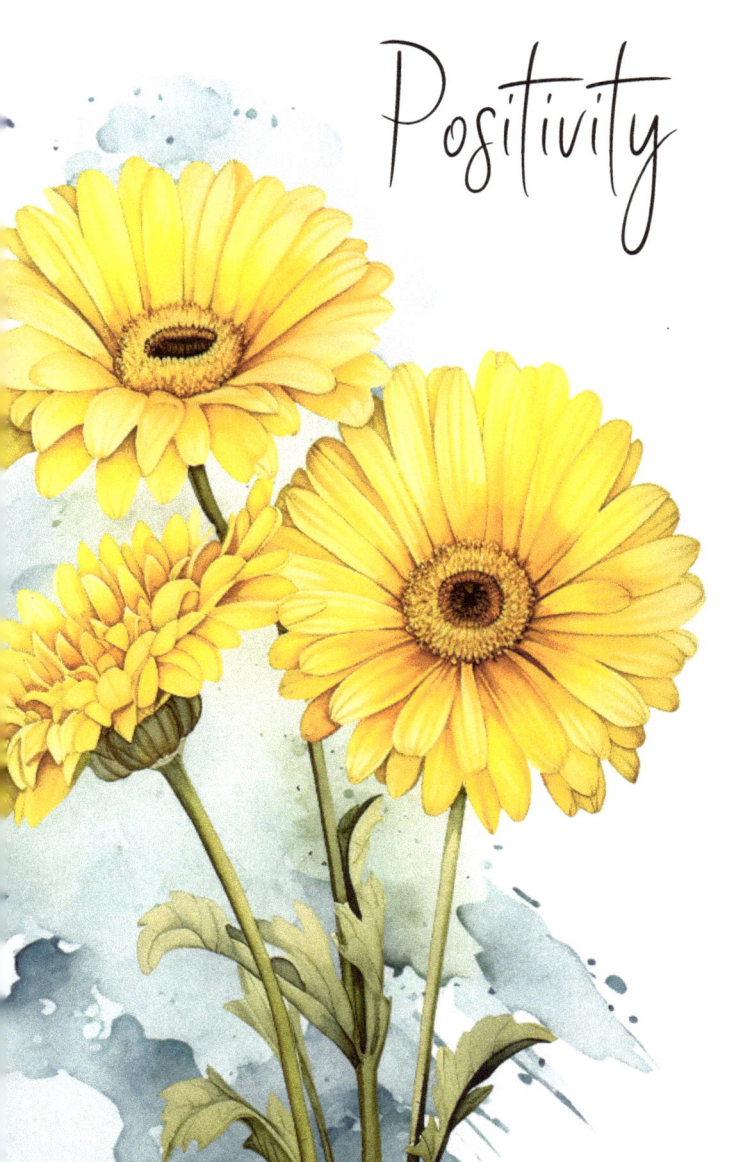

I trusted the wrong people,
that does not mean my
thinking is flawed.

When I hear something negative, I will think about something positive instead.

I acknowledge that toxic
people are not worth my time
or energy

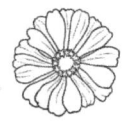

I will not be derailed by
negative people or situations.

I made some poor decisions, that does not mean that I am unable to change.

I am the only person here that can control my emotions

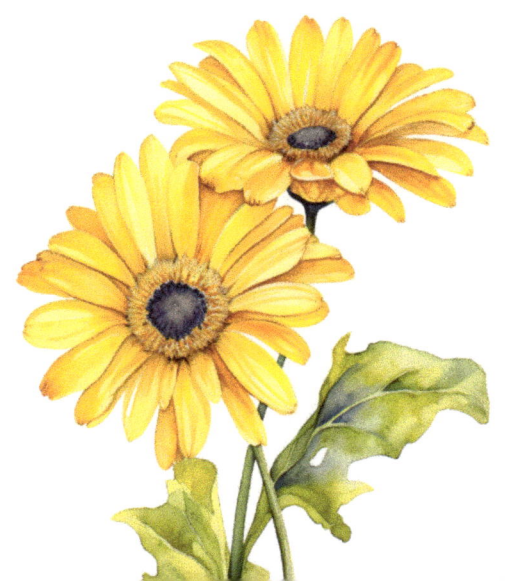

I will focus on my goals and dreams rather than the toxicity around me.

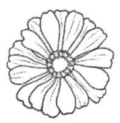

I recognize the beauty around me, even when I am in the presence of toxic people

Trusting people that lied to me is a reflection on them, and not a deficiency in me.

I am grateful for the good people and that is all that matters.

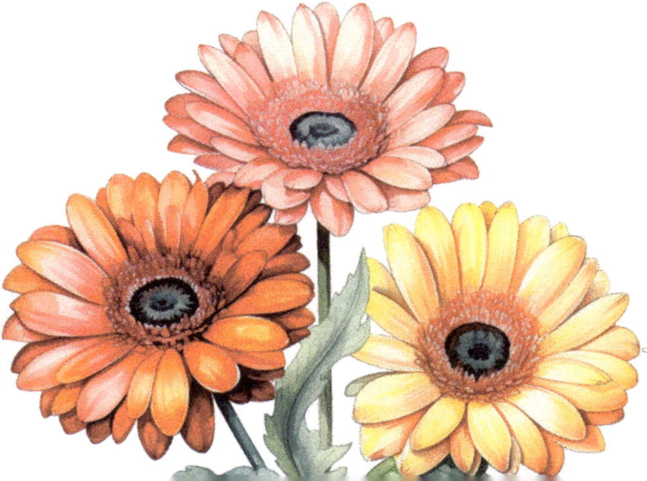

My past does not define me,
but it does allow me to change
and grow.

I will keep an open mind and focus on positive things

I choose to be joyful and optimistic.

I am powerful, and no one can take that away from me.

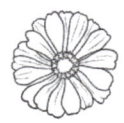

I am happy and positive.
No one can take that from me.

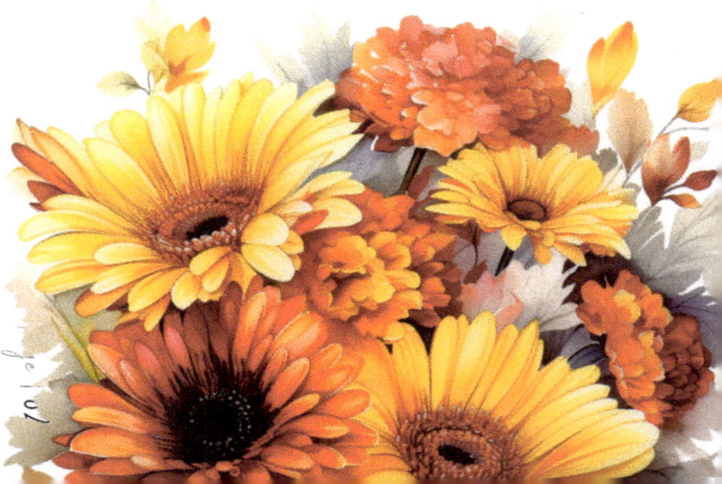

I will use difficult situations as a learning opportunity for what I do not want to be.

I know my worth and acknowledge that I am valuable.

I can choose the people I want in my life

I am committed to the boundaries I have set

I am proactive about managing the energy around me

I will only surround myself with people that support and uplift me.

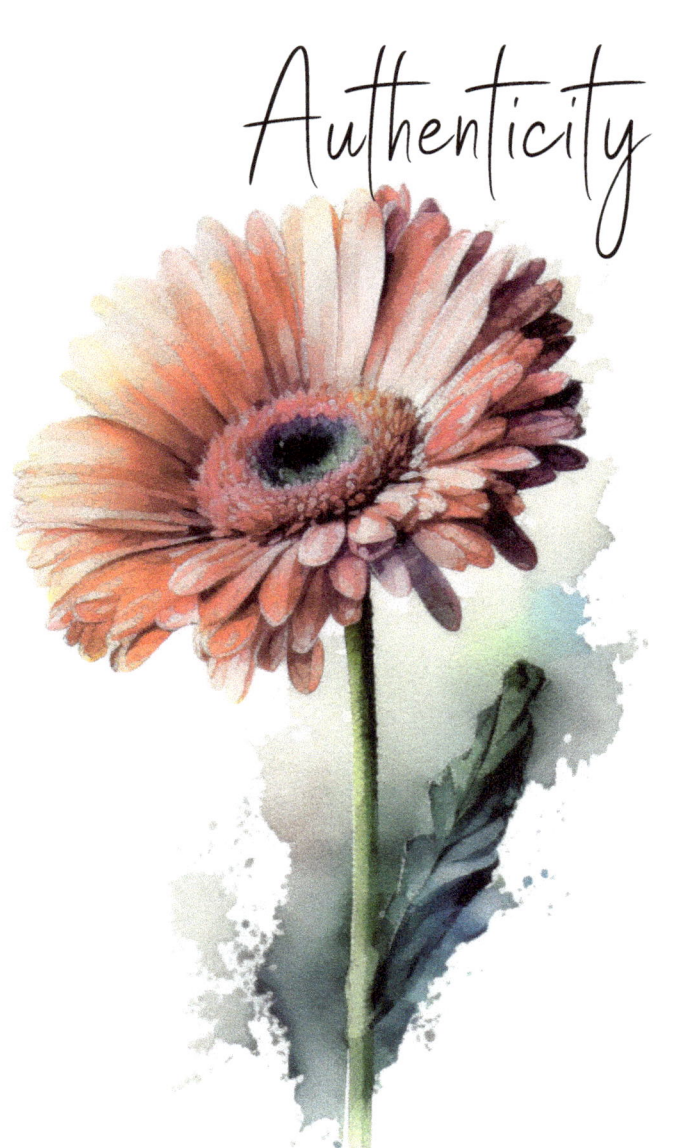

Authenticity

I will be real.

I will cry.

I will be angry,

I will be happy.

Being genuine is being yourself

I will not feel bad for cutting off people that show no remorse for hurting me

I will offer the best version of myself because that is my personal standard, even if I am frustrated or annoyed.

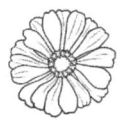

I will treat everyone with respect, even when it is challenging to do so

My behaviour and my choices are on me.

I am responsible for them.

Their behaviour and choices are on them.

I am not responsible for them.

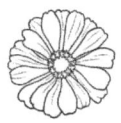

I will see what people show me who they are, not what they say.

Seeing good in people while they harm me is unhealthy.

I will no longer allow other people to cause chaos in my life.

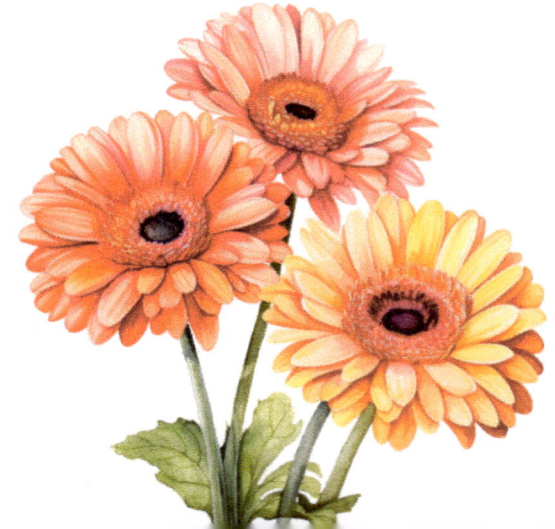

I am me.

Not the person others think I should be.

I am enough.

Emotions are expressing myself.

They make me human.

I will not take negative comments or behaviours personally.

When I hear something negative, I will think about something positive instead.

I will make the changes I need.
I am empowered to be the
positive influence

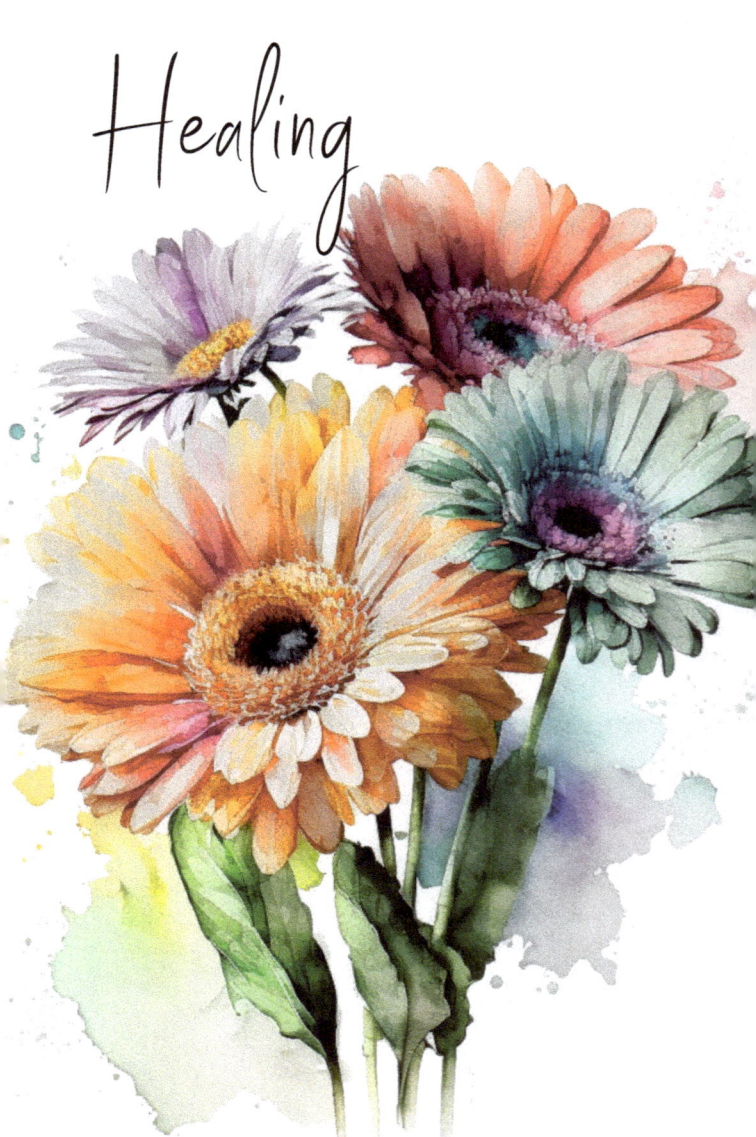

I chose to walk away and put my own happiness first.

I am saving myself.

I am not ashamed of my choice.

I am committed to finding something positive to focus on, even in negative situations

I am strong enough to choose
what is best for me

I needed a hero.

So that's what I became.

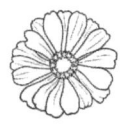

My life may be hard at times.

I may struggle, and I may stumble.

I will keep picking myself up and stay the course to find me.

I am strong.

I am capable.

I am me.

I know what I feel and why.

They are my emotions and my thoughts.

Only I know what I truly feel.

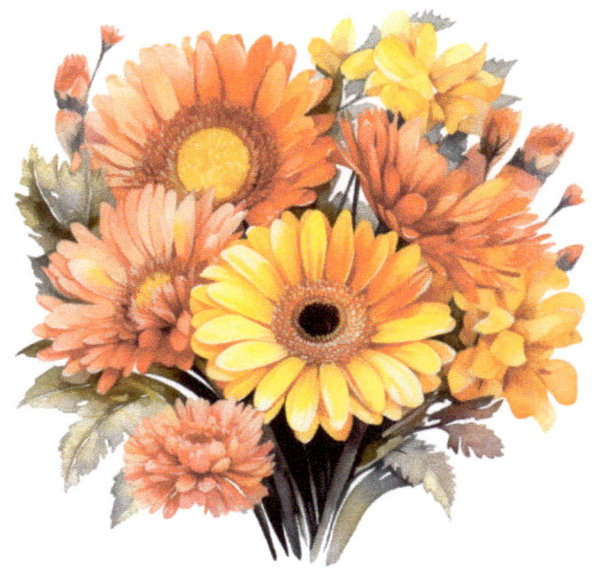

I love me.

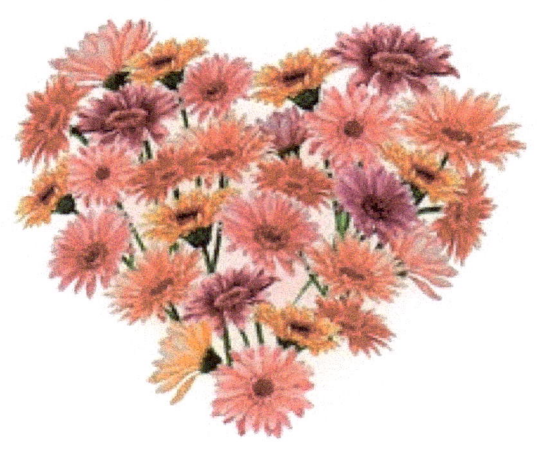

Look out for our other
affirmations books in the future:

Pink Rose
(Affirmations of Happiness)

White Chrysanthemum
(Affirmations of Truth)

www.ingramcontent.com/pod-product-compliance
Lightning Source LLC
Chambersburg PA
CBHW062040290426
44109CB00026B/2682